Table of Contents

ALS Hand Weakness Test - The Split Hand Index

1. Introduction to ALS and Hand Weakness

Focusing on the hands can be informative because often the hand with increased weakness may stay with a relatively normal small muscle movement due to a possible 'split' of the corticospinal neurons controlling finger movement. The hand experience may be reversed, often causing the stronger hand to be more likely to be the most weak when split is observed. At follow-up, the most affected side may experience an overall increase in the first dorsal interossei (FDI) muscle weakness despite a natural dominance of the abductor digit minimi in the control hand. Such an index might help determine the hand with greater muscle weakness, which is useful in assessing disease progression. In addition, that index can be used as an objective point to diagnose this symptom of hand weakness in studies of both new drugs to treat ALS and physiotherapy interventions to determine if they cause an improvement in hand muscle movement.

Amyotrophic lateral sclerosis (ALS) is a rare disease of motor neurons, a group of nerve cells that control the movements of the body. There are different types of motor neurons, including the corticospinal motor neurons that control the movement of the hands in response to signals from the brain. As these cells die in ALS, individuals notice weakness, stiffness, muscle wasting, and difficulty controlling finger movements. One of the first symptoms is difficulty performing tasks such as turning a key or buttoning a shirt. Definite diagnosis of ALS is not immediate because of the variety of symptoms, the length of time (up to a year) taken for the changes in the muscles to become obvious, and the rarity of the disease. It is important to be able to assess weakness in different muscles in a more objective way. Current trials of potential treatments have shown weaknesses in the current symptom scoring scales and strengths in new measurement tools that accurately assess the disease in these studies. Many scale developments study the hands due to the large burden of disease; hand disability is a major determinant of quality of life in ALS.

2. Overview of the Split Hand Index (SHI)

The Split Hand Index looks at the muscle atrophy in your hands and has four sub-indices. The tests in the thenar region – regarding the atrophy of the first dorsal interosseous (FDI) and abductor pollicis brevis (APB) branch of your median nerve (MN) – are used to evaluate the central change or the progression of the disease. The FDI muscle has been found to be affected earlier in the disease process than the APB. The amyotrophic lateral sclerosis functional rating scale (ALSFRS-R) only captures average scores in the FDI and does not evaluate the differences between the two muscles in the abductor pollicis tests. The hand weakness test also includes tests of the hypothenar muscle. In their published research article, Dr. Rutger Zietsma and his colleagues from Radboud UMC show how the hypothesis muscle differs based on motor neuron involvement in lower limb onset ALS.

The ALS Hand Weakness Test, also known as the Split Hand Index, is used to detect hand weakness and track its progression in ALS. "Split hand index" is more commonly used in scientific and research circles, but we'll refer to the test as the hand weakness test to make it easier to understand. Split hand index refers to the weakening of the thenar (asymmetrical) muscles in your hands while upper motor neurons continue to function normally in your hypothenar muscles. In our SHI subindex, two tests specifically target your thenar muscles. We also analyze your total SHI score, which observes the opposite movements to your hands and relates to muscle strength in your smaller hypothenar muscles.

3. Research and Development of the SHI

This paper is a scientific study developing a novel feature while using the Split Hand Index, the SHI, to assess patient hand weakness and predict negative and possibly even more important in small subpopulations, positive amyotrophic lateral sclerosis (ALS) diagnostic evidence. Many studies have examined the hand in ALS, with novel, precise function tests such as grip-force sensor-based strength monitoring, 3D motion capture devices and the Nintendo Wii Balance Board to measure static steadiness in the lower limbs and to a limited extent in the upper limb.

The restructured SHI retains the diagnostic advantages of the master formula but has advantages in practice and is easy to calculate. Concerning the SHI, the whole approach towards hand weakness has changed, and would be a good basis for further research, including in more homogeneous subpopulations such as upper motor neuron predominant ALS, theoretically producing a larger value, and lower motor neuron as the dominant clinical feature of progressive muscular atrophy (PMA). Both versions of the SHI could have some good advantages for the examination of patients with cognitive or swallowing deficits, when other data are not available. Further neurophysiological studies should be done in PMA subpopulations to better understand the nature of the split hand. A further advantage of both SHIs would be their ability to postdict ALS positives, providing a possibility for their inclusion into historical cohorts with long-term follow-up, a possibility that was not possible as the publication of the SHI in the article prior to this one.

4. Clinical Application of the SHI

"SHI can be a useful clinical tool for examining hand weakness in patients with ALS, and perhaps even other motor neuron diseases. Assess disease progression; predict enteral nutrition requirement, and relation to prognosis/survival. Assessment delineation of persons at higher risk to advance upper limb motor deficit. The level is especially affected when making a clinical decision, as limited evidence was found to support other quick and feasible clinical assessment measures. Nevertheless, SHI can impose a role in a 'real-world' patient setting by other healthcare professionals. Clinically, SHI plays a pivotal role in the assessment of dystonia for motor neuron disease, especially in corticobasal family disease with dystonia, and other dystonic hand disease. In a main recent study, for a definitive diagnosis of ALS according to revised EI Escorial Airlie House Criteria, SHI plays a role while including UEC despite lower motor neuron UMN conducted. In the same way, SHI classifies the disease segregation levels from having cognitive impairment in non-C9ALC72 to C9ALC72 patients. This can help differentiate between C9ALC72 and non-C9ALC72 patients using IRS without a cognitive viewpoint. SHI, by using an IRS cut-off score, is found to have some independent and joint utility when accounting for other demographic information to assist in categorizing patients into progression category levels. Product of time during the open phase and the SARA-IN score. Statistically, the model demonstrated a high degree of individual predisposition to this unique movement profile, as all patients displayed significant inter-patient variability in at least one SARA-IN subtask."

The effectiveness of the SHI lies in its ability to determine hand weakness. If a person is referred to me for evaluation of weakness, I can experience this weakness with my own two hands, but I must verbally report any difference in the ease of manipulation with my hands. The next time I see the patient in the clinic, it's possible that I will have my emotions confirmed by a quantitative score to document objectively the change that I subjectively detected at the initial visit. Such a measurement is helpful to a busy clinician but is also helpful for the patient.

The SHI can be a useful clinical tool for examining hand weakness in patients with ALS, and perhaps even other motor neuron diseases. As with any scientific tool, however, the real-world circumstances of the people who created the tool ought to be considered in its application. Dr. Sathi, a hand specialist (and not a movement disorders neurologist) trained by experts in using quantitative measures and forced to read all the papers on this subject for a series of lectures on the evaluation, diagnosis, and surgical treatment of patients with hand weakness.

5. Diagnostic Accuracy and Reliability of the SHI

In conclusion, the SHI has been reported to be an accurate diagnostic tool in the diagnosis of ALS hand weakness. Its reliability would be good if the measurement properties for testing between clinicians and, more critically, in an early motor neuron lesion population were less varied.

The diagnostic accuracy of the SHI was studied in a population with EMG proven MND in 2006. The published article suggested that, with over 96% predictive value, the SHI was of great value as a diagnostic tool. Internal control, in other words, the reliability of the SHI, was also proven to be consistent in a population of people who had their SHI repeated over a one-month period. However, recent work has assessed the reliability of the SHI over a six-monthly period, i.e., over a period of the condition deteriorating. Indeed, the SHI reported for 88% of within-clinician follow-up assessments were within 0.2 of one another, suggesting that the SHI has the capacity to be reliable as the condition progresses.

The Split Hand Index (SHI) has been suggested as the most beneficial tool in the diagnosis of ALS-related hand weakness at an early stage to facilitate early diagnosis, but also to allow for inclusion in a trial if required. Moreover, it is a helpful tool to monitor the disease. To utilize tools such as the SHI, they must be validated, i.e., checked for diagnostic accuracy and proven to be repeatable and consistent.

6. Comparison with Other ALS Hand Weakness Tests

Fatiguing tasks have been described in the Bailey, Kluin & Richards or in the Nine Hole Peg Test. However, they contain an important motor speed and coordination aspect. Comparison or correlation with these filigree tasks would not have been relevant. Instead, with force tasks, a correlation of increased force steadying with a more filigree task has been found: increased force steadying correlated with a decrease in coordination in short inclined target slide tests simulating icing sliding from under, in a slag flag test with a higher cognitive load correlated (negatively) with the shortened time taken to complete it. Yet another aspect of the SHI lies in the existence of an apparent optimal force for the AMT and in the quantification of faulty force control in each individual. The SHI represents a very complete tool that enables multiple aspects of hand function to be assessed.

Up to now, the introduction of the SHI completes the set of references to ALS hand and, even more specifically, finger functioning by introducing fatigability or finger irritation as a new concept. The design of the SHI has the particularity to distinguish between tasks using different muscle groups. Thus, its focus is partly different from tests like the Grooved Pegboard or Nine Hole Peg Test, which do contain an attention-demanding and fatiguing part.

Only a few references to hand functioning in ALS describe hand weakness using force tasks, such as grip force or pincer grip strength, etc.

7. Limitations and Future Directions

Since it is generally accepted that handedness should have more of a bearing on an ALS measure of hand strength than footedness, we assume that our decision to derive cut-off scores based on the dominant hand was appropriate for our pilot investigation. Other authors suggest that two SHI data outcomes could be used independently. However, this would considerably increase the number of collected data, resulting in increased time and human, systems, and statistical cost. Results collected at 10 centers serving a total of 39,000 patients registered on the Irish ALS Information Management System (AIMS) data demonstrate increased SHI/SHIN mean values with age (RH r=.329; LH r=.336; both p<.01) and marginally between males and females (RH p=.094; LH p=.071). Furthermore, SHI SHIN increases across 1st, 2nd, and 3rd quartile FVC (Kyphos) values. A parallel study aiming to help establish the feasibility and acceptability of this measure as a longitudinal marker of disease is currently underway in 47 of the 57 PCDN centers. A wider helped feasibility study across the entire PCDN is currently under review by 30 UK-based ethical review boards.

The Split Hand Index (SHI) appears to be a simple and well-tolerated tool and could be combined with other, more sensitive investigations to detect the critical phenotypic differences in ALS - C9orf72-ALS, TD-ALS, and LRS-ALS populations in future clinical trials and cross-sectional studies. However, it is known that ALS patient populations have variable rates of subsequent bilateral hand involvement. An estimation of immediate sequential progression is only possible where the split hand phenotype is present when the SHI is first performed in a newly diagnosed patient because it is known that those patients presenting with TDI less than 0.38 have an increased risk of rapid subsequent involvement of the contralateral hand.

8. Conclusion and Implications for Clinical Practice

Future studies need to determine SHI parameters to detect subclinical hand muscle weakness in patients with UMN signs compatible with primary lateral sclerosis. The findings of our study entail consequences for the daily practice of academic ALS centers and non-academic centers with a high interest in neuromuscular disorders. First, SHI cutoff values are helpful to see how slow or angularly the grip is deteriorating in ALS patients, which may have consequences for patient prognosis and the evaluation of treatment efficacy in drug trials, as a potential compensatory mechanism. Second, the analysis shows that grip force is decreasing in both the most affected hand as well as in the least affected hand, giving physiotherapists more arms and arguments to encourage the use of aids or ADL changes. This may improve the functional score at the least affected hand to identify disease progression in treatment trials. Third, our findings support the definition of limb onset and give an indication of the period between onset and first clinical signs in all ALS patients. This issue has become increasingly relevant since the first treatment for a treatable UMN phenotype (e.g., primary lateral sclerosis) has to be administered within the first two years of disease onset. Future prospective research needs to confirm these findings to result in stronger recommendations. Lower inter-rater reliability of the SHI than the grip force tasks might impede the implementation of the SHI in clinical practice.

This review summarized the psychometrics of the most commonly used tests to measure hand weakness in ALS. The conclusions predominantly stem from analyses of the last recordings. The extent of SHI development, extracted from those studies in which low unbiased values of SHI were recorded, suggests a development of SHI in about 1 year in limb onset and about 0.75 years in bulbar onset ALS patients, irrespective of the scoring system utilized. The most frequently used method (logarithmic grip strength) provided a cutoff value for ALS patients and HCs indicating SHI in a specific proportion of ALS patients (0.72-0.83 according to the used method). Yet, the SHI did not help in the diagnosis of ALS over other diagnostic tests. In short: given the results of this paper, I do not give preference to any specific SHI scoring system or SHI method diagnostic tool as none of them are able to have diagnostic superiority in the diagnosis of ALS.

The Diagnostic Value of Split Hand Index in Amyotrophic Lateral Sclerosis

1. Introduction

Amyotrophic lateral sclerosis (ALS) is characterized by the death of upper and lower motor neurons, leading to progressive muscle weakness and atrophy. Based on the clinical symptoms and the site of onset, patients can be classified into bulbar-onset and limb-onset ALS. Bulbar-onset ALS has a faster disease progression compared with limb-onset ALS. Both clinical nerve conduction studies (NCS) and electromyographical (EMG) examinations confirmed denervation activity, decreased throng motor unit action potential (MUAP) size, lesser collateral reinnervation and motor neuron loss involved in ALS showed great association with upper neuron degeneration. Statistics for potential biomarker tools for the diagnosis of ALS are shown in Supplementary Table S1. The results of EMG examinations are mainly divided into the denervated area and the only abundant area. The growth chain of EMG signals is from motor neurons to muscle fibers. The loss of motor units might result in masking, namely only abundant area surrounded the denervated units could be recorded when maximal voluntary contraction. Mimicking man might report an important index "pseudo-phase".

This study aimed to investigate the diagnostic value of the Split Hand Index (SHI), a new motor unit index in ALS. The optimum cut-off point of the SHI and whether the SHI could be used to predict the prognosis for those with ALS were also analyzed. We retrospectively collected data from those diagnosed with ALS according to both EI Escorial and

Awaji criteria between 2013 and 2021. Functional, neurological, and electrophysiological assessments were performed. Student's t-test, one-way ANOVA, and chi-square tests were used to compare differences between groups. The SHI showed a higher sensitivity and diagnostic accuracy and was able to be used for the early diagnosis of bulbar-onset ALS. Additionally, a cut-off value of 0.496 significantly separated those with ALS from healthy controls.

1.1. Background of Amyotrophic Lateral Sclerosis (ALS)

The split hand index is a true phenomenon in ALS in which thenar muscles are more severely affected. The dynamic study concerning the split hand phenomenon within the ALS disease course suggests that the pathological process mainly lies within the central nervous system. More attention should be paid to the relation between the clinical features and "split in reference to the lumbrical: interossei" instead of "split in reference to intrinsic muscles innervated by different nerves", since the atrophy of FDI might be a good surrogate biomarker of clinical severity in the absence of hand dysfunction in ALS.

Amyotrophic lateral sclerosis (ALS) is a fatal, progressive motor neuron disease that is characterized by degeneration of both the upper motor neuron and the lower motor neuron in the brain, brain stem, and spinal cord. The diagnosis of ALS is based on the revised El Escorial criteria, which provide to a certain extent the uniformity of the population enrolled in clinical trials and minimize the heterogeneity in the observed effect size. However, because of these strict criteria, about 10% of ALS patients have been classified as either clinical LMN with laboratory-supported UMNL (clinically possible ALS) or as laboratory-supported ALS who do not fulfill the clinical criteria of all-UMN frontotemporal dementia (clinically probable ALS). Thus, there is a need to develop simple and practicable new evaluation tools for ALS diagnosis. The split hand index was constructed on the premise that ALS preferentially affects the cortical motor neuron innervating the thenar eminence muscle (digit 1 muscles) more than those hand muscles without cortical representation. Mounting evidence now indicates that it is a true phenomenon, acquaintance of an abrupt thenar weakness and/or tremor is among the first motor features in ALS.

1.2. Significance of Early Diagnosis in ALS

One of the proposed diagnostic methods of ALS put forward by different researchers is the pathophysiological criterion of the Split Hand Index (SI). This term is understood as the relative reduction in thenar muscle strength in only one abductor pollicis brevis muscle with respect to abductor digiti minimi, resulting from an exaggerated preferential wasting of the FDI in ALS. This introduction proposes an overview on corticospinal system and the muscular effect of selective FDI reduction, the proposed mechanical model of SI, the finding of SI in ALS patients and its sensitivity and specificity as a diagnostic marker, and the association of SI to ALS severity and progression rate.

Through the years, early diagnosis of ALS has led clinicians to consider ALS as a potential therapeutic model for neurological diseases. A more accurate assessment of the patient with ALS might facilitate the most appropriate management and implementation of useful treatment strategies in resource allocation.

Early diagnosis of ALS brings indirect advantages, as it distinguishes patients with ALS from those with other neuromuscular and neurological diseases, allowing clinicians to more accurately disseminate information on prognosis and candidates for participation in clinical trials to patients and their families. ALS is a disease with a poor prognosis, and its neurodegenerative qualities mean it is important that diagnosis and the introduction of therapeutic interventions occur as soon as possible.

On one hand, patients who are still in doubt regarding the causes of their symptoms may seek additional opinions from different healthcare providers in order to find a true diagnosis, either delaying or proposing a delay in examination at the ALS clinic, thus losing time to optimize resources for the patients' care. Indeed, this fact is also responsible for other harmful consequences, such as losing valuable time with families and gradually losing independence to organize everyday activities or being forced into early retirement.

Amyotrophic lateral sclerosis (ALS) is a rapidly progressing, fatal neurodegenerative disorder which is diagnosed through exclusion of other disease types. As a result, several months from the onset of symptoms pass before receiving a definitive diagnosis.

2. Clinical Features of ALS

A few clinical features of ALS could be developed during the median follow-up of 343 or 392 or 597 days: dyspnea in a minimum of 46% of the subjects, intentional and unintentional weight loss in a minimum of 13.9%, fatigue in a minimum of 18.2%, and dysphagia in a minimum of 37% of the subjects. Objective measurement of fatigue in ALS in real life has no report in the literature. In the present study, the usage of SHI, which is the dystonic extension hand position, in the head rotation and elevated arm test and special task, could increase the accuracy of diagnosing ALS.

Clinical features of ALS are, however, nonspecific for ALS. They are very valuable for the differential diagnosis of similar diseases like primary muscular atrophy, primary lateral sclerosis, multisystem atrophy, multiple sclerosis, and Kennedy disease in subjects with progressive muscle weakness and spasticity. The utilization of some clinical features, diagnostic criteria, and EMG pattern of ALS has no importance in providing a mature diagnosis, especially in the early period and for the predictors of survival. The abbreviation of the split hand index (SHI) consists of the progression and timing relationship of the ulnar (lumbrical) and thenar region of the hand muscles of the dominant arm, to diaphragm, bulbar, and other hand muscles.

Amyotrophic lateral sclerosis (ALS) could be idiopathic or inherited. It is an upper motor neuron (UMN) disease and lower motor neuron (LMN) disease. The first symptoms are mostly progressing weakness or spasticity of the lower limbs or upper limb. Weakness of the distal muscle groups, atrophy, and fasciculation are seen in the upper extremity. Symmetric involvement of the corticospinal and bulbar tract is seen in this indispensable, fatal disease. The incidence of ALS is 2–5/100,000 person/year and the average life expectancy is 5 years.

2.1. Motor Symptoms in ALS

Poor hand function is typically reported among ALS patients for weakness. Although it is possible to reveal hand weakness with a simple dynamometer, hand involvement can be put forward in ALS patients without revealing the presence of weakness or at the earliest stages of the disease. MRC Grades developed to evaluate muscle strength provide moderate and volume-dependent reliability in evaluating early muscle weakness. In the case of pedunculoperoneal hypoglossal disease, loss of small diameter a-motor neurons can be detected before the loss of the larger diameter a-motor neurons decreasing the split hand sensory-motor index, which shows the severity of the difference between the abductor pollicis brevis and the first dorsal interosseous muscles. Similarly, in diseases such as ALS that cause peripheral denervation, the regression of large diameter muscle fibers is faster than the regression of small diameter muscle fibers due to current pathophysiological knowledge.

The main symptoms of amyotrophic lateral sclerosis (ALS), a neurodegenerative disease of adulthood, are loss of motor neurons in the brain and spinal cord. The disease progresses with muscle paralysis, and within an average of 2-3 years from the onset of complaints, motor neuron lesions lead to a state of disablement due to respiratory muscle paralysis or death. The disease starts in the extremities of the fingers or feet, sometimes drops floating around joints, and then gradually progresses through the limbs to the bulbar or chest muscles. Patients can also be represented with initial bulbar symptoms, sometimes with deglutition and speech problems. Loss of muscle mass, fasciculations, and paradoxical soft reflexes are the primary motor findings of the disease. In the early stages of the disease, the overlap of upper and lower motor findings in the same region helps to move to the direction of ALS.

2.2. Specific Hand Weakness in ALS

Distal hand muscle atrophy is commonly seen and reported as a "split hand" phenomenon in ALS. Weak specific hand muscles are observed and reported as a predictor of faster progression of ALS, like the key pinch and 3-point chuck pinch. However, the correlation is often less optimal. The adductor pollicis, first dorsal interosseous, and thenar muscles are distinctive muscles that also show scarce or no involvement in similar diseases such as polyneuropathy and multifocal motor neuropathy. The ulnar-innervated hypothenar muscle is not predominantly affected in other disorders that clinically resemble ALS. This specific pattern of weakness of hand muscles offers a high specificity for the diagnosis as well as progression of amyotrophic lateral sclerosis.

Pickels et al. indicated that patients with ALS present with specific patterns of weakness and wasting of intrinsic hand muscles, distinct from muscles that originate from structures at a more proximal level. This phenomenon, with a preference for distal muscles over proximal muscles in the hands, has been defined as the "split hand dysfunction" and has been made responsible for disturbing precision grip force. This distinct type of hand-related problem is a major determinant in the diagnosis of ALS after thorough clinical examination, especially when clinical examinations are combined with electrophysiological testing.

3. Split Hand Index

It is well known that several promising new biomarkers have emerged, and although there is still a long way to go before they can be implemented in routine clinical use, very large multinational clinical studies have already validated these new insights into the amyotrophic lateral sclerosis diagnostic process. Clinical tests in the field, such as the Split Hand Index, lateral spread reflex, cough bulbar function and fasciculation, are used to diagnose amyotrophic lateral sclerosis in clinical diagnostics. It is our intention to highlight the importance of the Split Hand Index in diagnosing amyotrophic lateral sclerosis in this article.

The Split Hand Index has been defined in recent years. It is calculated using MUNIX technique values of the abductor pollicis brevis (APB) and thenar compound muscle action potential (CMAP) obtained from conventional neurophysiological studies. The Split Hand Index represents a clinical reflection of the selective vulnerability of motor thenar/hypothenar muscles in patients with cervical spondylotic amyotrophy and ALS patients in neurophysiological testing. The split hand index is defined as follows in the first reports: ((MUNIX abd-2)/MUNIX abd) - (thenar CMAP/abd CMAP), where "abd" is abductor digiti minimi, "abd-2" is an MUNIX value from the abductor digiti minimi muscle at the second examination, "MUNIX abd" is an MUNIX value from the abductor digiti minimi muscle, and "thenar CMAP" is a compound muscle action potential from the thenar and hypothenar.

3.1. Definition and Calculation

Diagnostic Value of SI in the Literature: The split hand is very common in ALS, with a mean SI of 116.3 ± 7.2 in the entire group. Though SI has a rather high diagnostic value in the individual patient for ALS, the observation of an index value slightly above the upper limit can be caused by other diseases than ALS. Though SI is a diagnostic parameter with high potential to detect the presence of ALS, its value to confirm the disease in early phase is limited when going from the individual to the patient population, as indicated by a moderate likelihood of ALS expressed by the DOR. Anyway, our findings suggest the use of SI in the algorithm that includes neurophysiology in the diagnostic workup of patients with upper limb weakness of suspected lower motor neuron origin, taking into account consideration also to fib and MUNE.

Calculation: SI is defined as the mean of the percent actual bolus/bil standard deviation of the clinical dose mean value from the clinical mean area, expressed in percentage. SI = mean[(meanBolusCln/meanBolusbil) - 0.95 oh(EBolusCln/EBolusbil)] × 100.

Definition: Split-hand is a kind of neuropathy that is characterized by selective atrophy and weakness of the thenar/hypothenar muscles, relative to the muscles in the distal part of the upper limb. Split Hand Index (SI) is a measure for differential involvement of the thenar and hypothenar area relative to the more distal part in symptomatic motor neuron disease. SI is able to assess split hand status in many diseases by the very simple/most applicable formula of thenar/hypothenar muscle percent mean score, on a 0 to 4 scale.

3.2. Clinical Relevance

The findings from our studies revealed greater neurophysiological alterations in the LInd as well as greater electrophysiological impairment in the LInd at disease onset, during the early stages of the disease, and further throughout the disease in comparison to the ULInd/R abdomen, OLInd/T chin/ULInd/F regions. The impairment of single thenar muscles, as depicted by the forehead Split Hand Index (FH-SHI), differentiates rigorously between patients with ALS from healthy subjects. Multiple clinical utilities have been discovered regarding the diagnostic potency of SHI in the context of ALS, including data concerning the disease period.

Amyotrophic lateral sclerosis (ALS) is a relentlessly progressing neurodegenerative disorder primarily affecting motor pathways in the central nervous system. Characterized by the rapid loss of upper and lower motor neurons, patients usually die within 2-5 years after symptom onset, largely due to progressive paresis of respiratory muscles. While the diagnostic process depends mainly on the clinical assessment and investigation of neurophysiologic data, patients with ALS often encounter long delays before reaching their diagnosis. This delay may compound anxiety about potential medical conditions prior to receiving their ALS diagnosis. To accelerate the diagnostic process and provide patients with rapid, certainty-driven, and appropriate medical advice and care, feasible, alternative, valid, and specific diagnostic methods must be developed.

4. Diagnostic Criteria for ALS

According to the 2015 World Federation of Neurology Consensus, suspected ALS patients are defined on the basis of the presence of the relevant signs or symptoms of combined upper motor neuron (UMN) degeneration, lower motor neuron (LMN) degeneration and electrophysiological studies. To diagnose ALS, patients with symptoms of both UMN and LMN symptoms or signs must undergo further evaluation to make sure that it can be confirmed disease progression of the UMNs and LMNs, by clinical and electrophysiological evidence. According to the consensus of ALS in 2021, the diagnostic criteria of definite ALS in the early age of onset (EAO) and juvenile-onset ALS are determined according to the A1/B2 level as T1 C1 C2 and the S B level for the A1/B3 level. These guidelines can be used in clinical assessment. UMN, upper motor neuron; LMN, lower motor neuron.

ALS is a neurodegenerative disease characterized by selective and progressive degeneration of both upper and lower motor neurons, ultimately leading to their destruction. In order to make a definitive diagnosis of ALS, the symptoms and signs based on the typical location and changes in the upper and lower motor neurons are confirmed by neurophysiological tests of both peripheral and central nervous systems. There are many variations of the El Escorial revisited criteria and Gold Coast criteria for the diagnosis of ALS that focus on the importance of neurophysiological evaluations. Al-Chalabi, Rivas provide guidelines for patients with a clinical diagnosis of ALS, which further details the evaluation of bulbar involvement and clinical diagnostic guidelines for patients with definite, probable or possible ALS.

4.1. El Escorial Criteria

However, the main disadvantage is that they may be time-consuming and sometimes cannot be definitively decided for many months after the development of symptoms. Earlier in the disease course, the vital deciding factor is the time for the onset of symptoms in different regions of the body. The earlier the diagnosis, the better the management of the disease. Quality of evidence: high; strength of recommendation: low. It follows that the progression of ALS symptoms, seen as spread and multifocal involvement, is considered to be the gold standard for the diagnosis of ALS. Furthermore, the diagnosis can be declared in the absence of confirmative signs if spontaneous fibrillation potentials, positive sharp waves, voluntary activity, or fasciculation is seen on EMG in the two regions, as per the suggestion by a few authors.

The diagnosis of ALS is mainly based on the El Escorial Criteria, published by the World Federation of Neurology. The three sets of clinical criteria (classical El Escorial, Airlie House modification, and the revised El Escorial) describe the disease progression as a pattern of spread of neurodegeneration in the central and peripheral nervous systems, and the time of observation for the declaration of deficits in the multifocal progression. The definition for upper motor neuron signs (UMN), lower motor neuron signs (LMN), and the time period of progression is clearly given in the guidelines. These criteria are still the mainstay of the diagnosis of ALS and have the strongest Level A evidence. They are the most comprehensive and well-established criteria available and are widely used across the world. Any research on ALS will include patients who qualify for the El Escorial Criteria only.

4.2. Revised El Escorial Criteria

However, there is one clinical presentation associated with two clinical findings that are particularly consistent with ALS but are not included in the El Escorial criteria: the phenomenon of the split hand or split forearm, referred to in this revised publication as "split-hand/forearm syndrome" (SHFS). This syndrome is considered a pattern of disease spread in neurodegeneration. It has been clearly demonstrated with large motor unit potentials (neurogenic-positive sharp-waves in EMGs) in all muscles of the limb, except for the first dorsal interosseous muscle and the extensor digitorum communis. Thus, the high clinical and electrophysiological prevalence of SHFS in the typical-predominant form of ALS could represent a crucial part of the autoimmune post-epitopic scale of the entire burden of neurodegeneration. Since ALS criteria are based on patient behavior, particularly voluntary participation, the only way to offer a blending of neurology, behavior, and causality in a less subjective way is to use the causality of suitable electrophysiology as the basis for a human/molecular-operational bedside definition of ALS. The SHFS-ALS index alone is able to characterize the olivopontocerebellar syndrome-evolved-predominant ALS patients with limb variation, mainly debuts, and therefore a greater life expectancy. The SHFS-ALS handle with unequal rates of upper motor neuron (UMN) and lower motor neuron (LMN) degeneration diagnosis itself is able to be useful on its own, even in this older and clinically milder mature form of ALS. An interesting check in a possible future improvement in the SHFS-ALS handle methodology is if the addition of CMCT could extend SHFS-ALS performance. The SHFS-ALS discovery itself is able to be useful on its own, even in this older and clinically milder mature form of ALS.

The revised El Escorial criteria for the diagnosis of amyotrophic lateral sclerosis (ALS) are often used in clinical studies to exclude other conditions and aid in differential diagnosis. In the revised criteria, the category known as possible ALS was removed in order to increase the sensitivity of the diagnostic process and reduce the time to diagnosis. However, the revised El Escorial criteria do not take into account the journey of patients from their initial decision to consult a neurologist to the neurological referral. Recently, an updated revision of the diagnostic accuracy of the traditional El Escorial criteria to rule out ALS was published. According to the diagnostic studies, we can define the following intervals: from the first clinical symptoms to the time of ulnar hand-onset (the first muscle involved), then the progression of upper limb symptoms, and the presence of pyramidal syndrome, which is a major point for the diagnosis of definite ALS.

5. Utility of Split Hand Index in ALS Diagnosis

A weakness of the studies involving SOD1 is small samples, but despite that, two studies found a positive correlation and high Area Under the Curve (AUC), and only one found a correlation, but the patients from the control group were heterogeneous. The correlation with UMN signs is a strength of the Split Hand Index; homogeneity in the control group does not seem to have any major effect (AUC: 0.85-0.93). The Split Hand Index measures the hand muscles' weakness in a way that overcomes the overrepresented APB in the thumb index guiding abductor pollicis brevis. The differences come in intrinsic hand muscles; abductor digiti minimi is predominantly innervated by the anterior interosseous, whereas the interossei and lumbricals are innervated by both the median and ulnar nerves. The addition of abductor digiti minimi strength diminishes the accuracy of the Split Hand Index to diagnose patients with ALS. Sufficient abductor digiti minimi strength decreases the correlation between APB and FDI strength differentially.

The Split Hand Index is defined as: (abductor pollicis brevis-1st dorsal interossei) / (abductor pollicis brevis), and an increased Split Hand Index can help to diagnose Amyotrophic Lateral Sclerosis (ALS) patients. This technique has been widely studied. Several studies have confirmed its usefulness in differentiating between ALS and mimickers. The earliest prospective study to evaluate the Split Hand Index as a diagnostic test estimated the sensitivity and specificity of increasing Split Hand Index to diagnose ALS among patients with moderate upper motor neuron disorder to 83% (95% CI [68, 93]) and 87% (95% CI [70, 96]), respectively. When teaching electromyography, ultrasound, or when valuable signs are not available, the Split Hand Index can be used.

5.1. Studies Investigating Split Hand Index

5.1.2. Materials and methods. Split Hand was operationalized and when one arm or leg or combination meeting research criteria of the main study was identified, manual muscle testing (MMT) was performed in additional muscle unit(s). In detail, additional "Split muscles" diotad were also identified in anodic muscle units. An identified Split limb got two SI(s). In both the theoretical split muscles (where the clinically maximum UMN signs were expected under research diagnostic criteria) and the practically identified split muscles (diotad and additional ones). Features that can improve the clinical signs of UMN degeneration in ALS described were the UMN-LMN incongruities and the peculiar wrist and finger extensor muscle (E) subgroup in testing. Split Hand (SH) Index was the mean measure of congruous and incongruous groups having the most normal UMN signs. Initial Emotional lability (EL), Upper motor neuron (UMN) on CIVP, UMN-lower motor neuron (LMN) discordance subgroup, and Disability (swallow, tongue). Longitudinally, for the survival analysis of groups, Initial EL was transferred to the Upper motor neuron (UMN) subgroup that derived the most strength drop in both longitudinal and the survival analysis.

5.1.1. What's already known? Split-hand index (SI) is a new measure to identify clinical upper motor neuron (UMN) impairment and differentiate ALS and mimics. Split hand phenomenon, a clinical sign related to motor cortical function, is becoming the new star in ALS. In ALS, other

UMN-including muscles in a myotomal area will catch up to the first affected muscle over time, facilitating the muscle strength retention that may occur. Some of the UMN-including first overlapping muscles are recruited diotad or beyond, making the upper motor neuronal signs disproportionately greater in already affected muscle unit(s) as compared to the muscles that are yet to be involved.

5.2. Limitations of Split Hand Index

Fluctuating clinical signs that are common in ALS could affect the results of the SHI. Daily functional hand capacities, such as grasping and pinching, are multifactorial and are influenced by several parameters. Finger temperature, tested in the lowest and heaviest members, the skin of these being partially implanted into cutaneous fatty tissue supplied by blood, is heavily susceptible to sympathovagal balance mediated by the autonomic nervous system. Sympathovagal balance is involved in emotional processing and is sensitive to stress. In acute stress like stage fright, hand skin temperature decreases robustly within minutes. Answers in skin blood flow are opposed to each other and in direct relation with anxiety level (higher tone gives a lower temperature in very cold-warm hands).

One of the main limitations is the cut-off values we use, which can modify the sensitivity and the specificity of the test. Cardiovascular damage caused by the disease, due to autonomic nervous system involvement, can modify the hand's temperature, the gap between the values, and the SHI itself. These variations potentiate subjects that will be negative in the test, probably in the earliest stages of the disease. We suggest the use of ST and FTCOG with their middle limit or also OPCG as additional measures to improve diagnostic accuracy. The combination of several signs or times of disease course allows for the detection of cabin degeneration in a single patient and can greatly improve the SHI accuracy. The use of skin temperature as a marker of autonomic involvement could assist in SHI interpretation.

Despite the utility of SHI, it has some limitations that hinder it from being used as a unique diagnostic tool.

5.2. Limitations of SHI

6. Conclusion

Diagnosis in early stages plays a key role in deciding the patients to be recruited to clinical trials. In the follow-up of the patients that magnetic stimulation cannot be performed because of later deceased, the decreases in SHI scores in line with muscle weakness assessed on manual muscle testing and neurophysiological tests with the course of the disease will be useful on the indication of lower motor neuron involvement in brachio-cervical region. Otherwise, knowing the predicted prognosis time and the presence of lower motor neuron involvement can have positive effects on disease management and guide therapeutic intervention. All of these will provide a significant contribution to clarify ALS pathology.

In summary, it can be concluded that the SHI can be used as a new, simple, noninvasive clinical test in the diagnosis of ALS. The SHI positively correlates with the AHSS and may show the severity of the disease. SHI values were significantly higher in patients with ALS compared to healthy controls and ALS mimicking diseases. This index can point to lower motor neuron involvement in the brachio-cervical region of patients with ALS. The SHI could be enquired and calculated retrospectively from the patient who cannot be examined due to passed. Future studies to be conducted prospectively on larger series including all phenotypes of ALS will facilitate the confirmation of this situation.

6.1. Summary of Key Points

The diagnostic value in distinguishing MND patients from healthy controls is best for SHI followed by AH. However, the highest diagnostic significance seems to concern the IB-ALS phenotype in the same comparison group (HC and OMND). Despite we tried to select qualifiers from comparison groups, the risk of bias or confusions is high and may affect the rapid translation of these preliminary results toward practical application. One of the limitations of the study is related to the fact that the sample size is relatively small, and a larger series of patients should be studied in the future. In addition, future studies should take into consideration including CMT and HNPP patients in the control group.

The Split Hand Index (SHI) may have an important diagnostic value in a specific population of patients with motor neuron impairment. Therefore, SHI could be useful in differentiating between ALS patients and HC, MND mimics, and other neurodegenerative patients. This parameter does not depend on the severity of weakness of the thenar and hypothenar muscles or the AH in ALS patients, and therefore, it is stable over time, which corrects the deficiency in another commonly used parameter, the thenar index (TI), which is not stable. The values of SHI of patients with IB and PMA as ALS phenotypes were significantly higher compared to HCs, MND mimics, and other neurodegenerative patients.

6.2. Future Directions in ALS Diagnosis

A novel diagnostic criteria utilizing natural history data (MRITB, MRITB-ALS) showed substantial agreement (κ = 0.755) between a clinician-based diagnosis of ALS and diagnosis via an algorithm derived from a model that included total, lower limb, and diaphragm MRI T1-w TI at baseline and their rates of change over time. Further studies incorporating other diagnostic measures and larger patient cohorts are warranted. As the understanding of MND continues to explore different manifestations and pathways in this complex disease, improvements can be made to the diagnostic criteria to better capture the diagnostic trajectories of this condition. Future studies can focus on evaluating the applications and clinical relevancy of using SpHI in current or other overlapping clinical settings or natural history studies of non-symptomatic PwMND. In the future, the use of the natural history SpHI in diagnostic criteria may help to distinguish cut-offs and build consensus to help define diagnostic criteria for PwMND.

To date, the SpHI has been evaluated as a diagnostic tool for MND in people who are experiencing symptoms and deficits, which would not be sufficient evidence alone to make a diagnosis of MND because of the similar motor impairments often seen in radiculopathies. A study evaluating SpHI values in non-symptomatic to differentiate them from symptomatic PwMND (who presented to a neurology clinic with bulbar or upper limb impairments that were concerning for MND), will be informative to evaluate the utility of the SpHI to diagnose MND in clinical practice. There is emerging evidence for diagnostic techniques in ALS such as quantitative MRI and muscle ultrasound. For these, there is potential to use these to contribute to diagnosing PwALS in the future, beyond neurophysiological and clinical assessments. The SpHI predicted faster progression of ALSFRS-r (respiratory subscore/mo), and shorter survival time.

www.ingramcontent.com/pod-product-compliance
Lightning Source LLC
Chambersburg PA
CBHW071123260726
48661CB00006B/2683